NO GREATER LOVE

"All of Christ's faithful,
whatever be the conditions, duties,
and circumstances of their lives,
will grow in holiness day by day
through these very situations..."

Vatican II: Constitution on the Church, 41

JOHN MILSOME

NO GREATER LOVE

Damien, apostle of the lepers

St Paul Publications

St Paul Publications
Middlegreen, Slough SL3 6BT, England

Cover design: Mary Lou Winters FSP
Maps: Elissa Vial
Printed by the Society of St Paul, Slough
ISBN 085439 308 0

St Paul Publications is an activity of the priests and brothers of the Society of St Paul who proclaim the Gospel through the media of social communication

Contents

For my wife Isobel
for all her help on this book

Introduction

This is the story of a man who devoted his life to the welfare of lepers on the island of Molokai in the Pacific Ocean. The name of the man was Joseph de Veuster, better known as Father Damien.

Leprosy is a disease found mostly in tropical countries. We can read of it in the Bible but it was not until the fifth century AD that leprosy came to Britain. There were lepers living as outcasts in Saxon and Norman times and their numbers increased during the years of the Crusades.

During the reign of Edward III they were not allowed to enter London but were sent to special homes called Lazar houses. Here they were given a stick, clothing and a bell or wooden clappers to warn others of their approach. Despised and feared by everyone, they could only obtain food by begging.

Then, in 1119, help came from an order of monks known as the Knights of St Lazarus. They built homes called lazarettos where the lepers could stay and be assured of friendship, kindness and help. After the terrible plague called the Black Death in the fourteenth century, few lepers survived and the lazarettos were closed.

There are still millions of lepers in the world today but they receive help through the United Nations. In Burma, for example, at least 200,000 were given sulphone drugs and other treatment. This gave the patients hope that their condition could be arrested and might well improve.

When Father Damien arrived in Molokai, he found daunting conditions. People were scared to come to help the lepers who therefore had neither doctors nor nurses. The hospitals on the island were just places where lepers in the late stages of the disease went to die. He found too that many of them were living in a terrible state of hunger and squalor and misery.

Damien was a foreigner and some of the lepers initially were suspicious of him and did not make him welcome. By his own example of hard work, sense of purpose and the ability to inspire hope, he won them over as friends. His life was a wonderful example of self-sacrifice and dedication by one human being for others who needed help so desperately.

Father Damien had no special advantages in life except a strong character and great determination. The way he created hope and even happiness in the leper colony eventually made both himself and Molokai world famous. In the end, his toil among the lepers brought the inevitable, and the customary opening words of his sermons, "We lepers", were no longer simply a spiritual sharing in their affliction.

He carried on his work for nearly four years after the diagnosis of leprosy, and died on 15th April 1889.

He would have been glad to know that today,

Christians throughout the world are still working for lepers. Especially would he have been delighted that modern surgery and drugs such as dapsone can arrest the disease and help lepers to be rehabilitated back into society.

1

"Here I am, Lord"

Joseph de Veuster was born on 3rd January 1840, at Tremeloo in Belgium. He was a lively child. One of his tricks was to jump on the back of a horse-drawn cart as it trundled by. Encouraged by the shouts of the other children, Joseph would hang on as long as he could. Then he would jump clear, hoping the driver had not seen him. In winter he loved to skate on the frozen waterways.

In the evenings Joseph enjoyed sitting by the fire with his brothers and sisters while their mother read to them from a large volume of lives of the saints. The children listened carefully and were fascinated by what they heard. They were quick to notice that the saints often went away to deserts to think and pray. So exciting did the children find the stories that they made up their minds to try and live like hermits themselves.

There were no deserts near Tremeloo, of course, so the children decided one morning to go to a nearby woodland. Here they knelt down under the trees and talked about the saints. They all agreed that they should lead a life of quiet thought and then they said their prayers. They were still there in the evening when a man from the village saw them. He stopped to question them, wondering what they could be doing away from their homes after sunset. When he realized that they were the De Veuster children he took them home at once.

Joseph's love of prayer grew throughout his childhood. On one occasion he could not be found anywhere in Tremeloo and his family became anxious. It so happened that, not far away, there was a fair which attracted people from miles around. But, the missing boy was not to be found at the fair. He was eventually discovered at prayer in the nearby church away from the noise and jostling crowds. The village school, with its untrained school-teacher, provided only the rudiments of education. When he left school Joseph worked with his father in the fields. As always, he worked very hard and was willing to try his hand at everything. In what little spare time he had after a hard day on the farm, he always seemed to be studying books. This made his parents believe that he was capable of benefiting from opportunities of higher education.

Joseph spoke Flemish but his French was not so good. His parents therefore decided to send him to a school in Braine-le-Comte which was in a Walloon or French-speaking part of Belgium. He was by no means brilliantly clever but his capacity for sheer hard work enabled him to achieve good standards.

All the time he was thinking about his future and felt drawn to follow his elder brother, Auguste, into the religious life. There was much to consider – his parents needed his help on the farm. Possibly

Joseph would have spent his life as a farm-worker if his father had not needed to go, one day in 1858, to Louvain to transact some business and suggested to Joseph that he might like to accompany him. It was agreed that while there, Joseph should visit Auguste, who had joined the Congregation of the Sacred Hearts of Jesus and Mary. Around this time Joseph found he could no longer resist the inner longing to enter the religious life. He decided to apply for admission to the same Congregation as his brother. He was duly accepted and his parents respected his decision. Lacking the necessary education to be admitted as a student for the priesthood, Joseph had to enter as a lay brother and this he did early in 1859.

On entering the religious life Auguste had taken the name of Pamphile. When Joseph entered he took the name of Damien. Damien's enthusiasm for learning led Pamphile to teach him Latin. The progress made was such that, after several months, Damien's superiors were sufficiently impressed to allow him to change his status and become a student for the priesthood.

Damien's studies were nearing completion when Pamphile was selected to be among a group of missionaries being sent to the Hawaiian Islands (or Sandwich Islands as they were then known). Damien hoped fervently that such an opportunity would one day be his. Throughout his student days he had frequently prayed before a picture of St Francis Xavier, the great Jesuit missionary, that he would be sent out on the missions.

Shortly before he was due to depart Pamphile caught typhus and clearly was not going to be well enough to sail on the appointed date. Damien understood his brother's disappointment. He asked him if there was any chance that he could go in his place. Pamphile said that, although it was only a faint chance, he should write to the Superior General. Damien wrote, more in hope than with confidence. Days later a letter arrived for him from Paris. To his surprise and delight Damien found that his name had been included in the chosen list of missionaries for the Sandwich Islands.

Towards the end of October 1863 Damien set off, with the other missionaries, for Bremerhaven from where they began their long and hazardous voyage to Honolulu. From the ship, Damien wrote to his family: "We have very small cabins in which there are two berths placed one above the other. Our life on board will be as if we were in a monastery; we shall keep the same rules as at Louvain. We shall have hours for prayer, study and recreation in the saloon which serves as a refectory and for all else we have to do."

During the five months at sea there were violent storms which, fortunately, the ship survived. After rounding the Cape of Good Hope, they sailed into a storm of great ferocity. For two weeks the ship was battered by gales and giant waves. Damien did what he could to help those who were sea-sick and, when extra hands were needed on deck, he worked alongside the seamen, handling the ropes and sails.

Apart from the storms there was the great heat to contend with and the monotony of the food that had to be endured day after day. The tiny cabins were uncomfortable and stuffy and, even on deck, the stench from the ship's hold was hard to bear. It was a great relief to the travellers when they saw their destination in the distance.

They landed on 19th March 1864. Damien was sent to a college near Honolulu to prepare for his ordination to the priesthood, two months later.

He wrote to Pamphile about the event and about offering his first Mass: "Recall the feelings you yourself experienced, the day you had the happiness of standing at the altar for the first time. Mine were the same with this difference, that you were surrounded by friends and brothers in religion, while I was surrounded by children, recent converts, who had come from all parts to see their new spiritual fathers... Strong were the emotions I experienced in giving, for the first time, the Bread of Life to a hundred persons, many of whom had, perhaps, been on their knees before their ancient gods."

Soon afterwards Damien was appointed by the Bishop to work in the Puna district of Hawaii. As the Bishop was going to Hawaii to bless a church Damien was able to travel with him. They set off in early June by steamer. On the way, the boat called at the island of Maui and Damien was delighted that they were able to visit the missionaries there, albeit briefly. As the steamer left Maui there was nearly a disaster. Damien later wrote home and described what happened: "We had hardly left the harbour when the ship caught fire. There was just time to extinguish it before the wood was burnt through, so the water did not get in. We turned back immediately and once more found ourselves safe and sound at the house of our father of Maui."

Damien relished the opportunity this mishap had provided of gaining more valuable advice and information from the experienced missionaries. So taken up was he with this that he was not on hand when the next steamer arrived, and the Bishop went on without him. Damien had to wait until the original steamer had been repaired, two weeks later, and then set off in the Bishop's footsteps eventually catching up with him on 24th July. It was just the beginning of much journeying on foot and horseback.

2

In the Lord's vineyard

Once Damien had settled into his life as a missionary, he wrote home to Belgium, giving his first impressions: "The climate is delightful, so that strangers easily become accustomed to it and generally enjoy better health here than in their own country. The archipelago is made up of eight islands, four of which are large and four small. Hawaii, the one on which I am stationed, is larger than all the others together. It is as large as Belgium, if not larger. In the centre are three volcanoes, two of which appear to be extinct. The third is still active, and it is in the neighbourhood of this that Providence has destined me to be placed. From one end of my district to another, you have to walk on lava."

Damien became a familiar sight as he travelled from village to village, making new friends and preaching. His great physical strength and stamina were very useful to him. It was exhausting, walking or riding in the dust and heat.

When he heard that a fellow-missionary, Father Clément Évrard, who looked after the much larger area of Kohala-Hamakua, was not physically fit enough to cope, Damien quickly asked to be allowed to exchange his district for the larger area. He was delighted when his request was granted.

The new area covered around 1,000 square miles, and it took Damien more than a month to go round it and see the people in all the villages. They were always glad to see what eventually became the familiar sight of Damien astride his horse with a loaded mule trotting beside them. He grew to love these people and never minded any personal hardship he had to endure to help them.

Parts of the area were so remote that it was impossible for him to reach them on horseback. He knew that somewhere on the other side of a high mountain there were people living in a village. He was determined to visit them, if it was at all possible. With the help of some island canoeists, he set out to find a beach that would enable him to go inland without climbing a mountain.

The sea was infested with sharks and the tides were treacherous for a small craft. The canoe was soon being tossed and turned in all directions and the islanders found it difficult to keep it under control. Suddenly a huge wave overturned the canoe. Damien and his crew were pitched into the sea. They swam towards the shore which fortunately was not too far away and, as they were strong swimmers, they managed to reach dry land.

In spite of this setback, Damien was determined to find a way of reaching the remote inland regions of his area. A week after the accident in the canoe he set out again. This time he went on horseback, riding in the direction of the mountain. He hoped to find tracks that he could follow inland. He had to travel alone and unaided for there was no guide to show him the way.

There were no roads but for four days he rode towards the mountain until at last he reached its slopes. Then the mountain track became so steep that his horse could not keep its footing. If it slipped and fell, both horse and rider could be seriously injured. Damien decided to leave the animal and go on alone.

He had to scramble up the mountain on his hands and knees until sheer exhaustion forced him to rest. Then on he went again, up and up towards the summit.

At last his strength and determination enabled him to reach the top where he found himself looking down on a steep ravine.

He was horrified to see how steep was the slope on the other side of the mountain. One false step and he could plunge into a ravine and fall thousands of feet to certain death. He had hoped that in the valley he would see signs of human habitation. There was no village in sight however, only wild countryside with a second mountain in the distance which looked as high as the one he had just climbed.

It would have been logical at this stage for Damien to have given up. But that was not his character. Once he started something, he had to see it through to the best of his ability. This time was no exception.

He began the slow, exhausting and dangerous task of descending into the valley. At last he reached level ground and began to make his way towards the next mountain, hoping that on the way he might come across a village that had not been visible from the mountain-top.

Unfortunately he saw no sign of either people or their houses.

With his boots nearly torn from his feet by the ragged, mountain rocks and his hands cut and bleeding through his constant stumbling on the uneven track, he reached the slopes of the next mountain. Even then he would not stop, but struggled to the top. Here, he rested for a while to look down once again into another valley.

It was a great disappointment when there was still no sign of human life. To add to his difficulties, clouds had come over the mountains and the weather was changing. Heavy rain poured down, making his progress a misery as he clambered over the wet and slippery rocks. He had come too far to think of turning back and could only stop for occasional shelter and rest, still hoping for the sight of a village.

Lashed by wind and rain, he somehow reached the second valley and began to climb the third mountain. There was no shelter for him to sleep so, although he was soaked to the skin and desperately tired, he found the strength to reach the summit of the third mountain. There must surely be people living somewhere near but there was still no sign of a village.

With his senses reeling, he went down the mountain and started to cross the valley. He felt so weary that he could hardly stand. Suddenly everything went black and he pitched forward on the ground, unable to rise.

Exactly how long he was unconscious he never knew, but he was aware of anxious faces looking down at him. Some islanders had found him and carried him to a stream where they moistened his mouth and face with water. When he was able to sit up and thank them, they explained that they were from the nearby village. Damien was delighted: the people he had been seeking had found him.

These friendly, hospitable people invited him to come and stay in their village and he, naturally, accepted. They had no church and Damien explained to them that now he had recovered he would like to repay them for their help by building them a place of worship. They were astonished to see the man they had thought was dead now busy chopping down trees and sawing and hammering the wood.

His great energy and determination was an example to all of them. The enthusiasm he showed was infectious and soon the villagers were wanting to help.

At last the chapel was finished and everyone gathered round to watch Damien complete the final task. He climbed proudly onto the top of the building to fix a large wooden cross to its gable.

Before leaving the village, Damien taught two Christian men to read lesson in the chapel, so that the people would have some spiritual help and comfort in the absence of a priest. Damien felt inspired by the warmth of their friendship and, successful though his visit to them had been, there was some sadness in his heart as he left them. He knew he was leaving a place that would be very difficult to come back to again, although he would certainly try.

It was a hard, adventurous life that he led. But, there were times when he suffered from the fact that contact with a fellow-priest was only possible every two or three months. He felt strongly that a missionary needed the help that came from the meeting with other missionaries.

His zeal for helping all who might need him never slackened. One day, he was walking on the beach when he saw a small boat drifting in the sea. Then he noticed men in the boat, slumped in strange positions and making no attempt to use their oars. Damien called to them but received no reply. He had no boat of his own but he was sure these people needed help. So he plunged into the sea and swam towards the boat which he reached safely.

On board were eight sailors whose ship had been wrecked. They had been in their small open boat for many days and nights. Their supplies of food and drink were now gone. Damien rowed them to the shore and, with the help of some of his island friends, carried them to his home. He gave them food and, as they recovered and were able to talk, he discovered that he had rescued four Englishmen, three Americans and a Dutchman.

For several days Damien welcomed them as his guests. They described how they had rowed day after day until exhaustion had left them at the mercy of the tides. Even when at last they sighted land, they were too weak to row. If it had not been for Damien, they might well have drifted far out to sea and died.

When the seamen had fully recovered they wanted to sail on to Honolulu. They watched for a sight of any passing boat. Eventually one appeared on the horizon and approached near enough for them to wave. In response to the signals, the boat stopped near the shore. The seamen thanked Damien for everything he had done for them and sailed away.

In 1867 the volcano erupted and Hawaii experienced some terrible earthquakes. Buildings fell as the ground opened up after shaking terrifyingly. During one violent earthquake hundreds of people were injured and thirty-one killed. The earth movements caused a great tidal wave which surged over the land, drowning more than forty of the islanders. Damien survived these dangers but was still mentioning the earthquake in letters to his parents a year later.

In his letters he often described his work, and

by 1868 was writing that he now had the welcome assistance of another priest who had come to the Kohala-Hamakua area. In one letter he wrote: "In the four years I have been here, I have built four new churches and repaired one old one. I myself had to do the work of a carpenter. I have still one or two chapels to build in my parish and then we can live more comfortably." He ended his letter by mentioning that there were lepers in Hawaii and that most of them were sent away to the island of Molokai.

Leprosy had been one of the most dreadful diseases known to mankind for thousands of years. Once a person became a leper nothing could be done to cure them and the illness became gradually worse until they died. Because leprosy was infectious and contagious, doctors were reluctant to help the victims. So, these unfortunate people were shunned and made to live apart from healthy people.

When it was decided to send all lepers to Molokai, there were miserable scenes as families were forced to say goodbye to their loved ones. The leper settlement was situated in a rocky, uninviting place, and when the writer, Robert Louis Stevenson, visited the island, he was horrified by what he saw. Later he wrote, "I am not a man more than usually timid but I never recall the days and nights I spent on that island promontory without heartfelt thanks that I am somewhere else."

The treatment of the lepers in Molokai greatly

troubled Damien. He witnessed the sadness as they had departed to face a future without any kind of help. Stories he heard about conditions in Molokai were not pleasant. Some lepers could work but others were not able to walk. There was cruelty, robbery and even murder.

In 1873 Damien went to the island of Maui to be present at the consecration of a new church. The Bishop who carried out the ceremony spoke of the problems of trying to cure leprosy and the help needed for lepers. He hoped there would be some priests who would have the courage to go and work on Molokai at the Kalawao leper settlement. The Bishop knew that anyone going to live permanently in the leper colony would almost certainly catch the disease. So, he did not appeal directly to any individual priests to make such a supreme sacrifice. He suggested to them that a rota might be arranged so that no priest would remain on Molokai for more than a few weeks at a time.

Damien immediately volunteered along with several other priests. It was agreed that Damien should be allowed to go first.

The boat on which the Bishop was to travel back to Honolulu was stopping at Molokai, on the way. And so, with no time for farewells, Damien set out with the Bishop on the boat which was also carrying a group of fifty lepers bound for Molokai.

When the Bishop and Damien landed, they were surrounded by a large crowd of lepers. The

Bishop spoke to them: "So far, my children, you have been left alone and uncared for, but you shall be uncared for no longer. I have brought you one who will be a father to you."

Soon it was time for the Bishop to say goodbye and return to Honolulu. As he watched the boat sail away, Damien knew that he was now quite alone to begin the great task of helping the leper community. It was to be his life's work and would make his name known the world over as the lepers' friend.

But, first he had to get accustomed to the sights and smells of leprosy.

Even worse than the lepers he saw walking about the village were those who could only lay in their huts. These were the really bad cases, so ill that they could not move from their beds. Some of them were living in conditions of squalor on their beds of leaves and twigs with no hope of getting better. He went to every hut and tried to find a word of encouragement for them all.

He saw some stone ruins. Out of curiosity he approached these to examine them carefully. Coming up to them through some bushes, he uttered an exclamation of surprise. Under the walls were what looked like dead bodies but then he noticed some were moving. A man came from the shadow of the walls and Damien asked him why these poor people were under the wall.

"They are lepers like myself," said the man. "But they are too weak to build a hut. I have a brother who lives here with his wife and every day I bring them food and water." In a few hours on Molokai, Damien saw more suffering than the vast majority of people see in a life-time.

Some months before Damien's arrival, one of the Brothers of the Sacred Hearts Congregation had built a small chapel at Kalawao. It was named after St Philomena. Damien made his way to the chapel, and found it in need of repair and very dirty inside. Here was something that Damien could remedy at once. He strode from the chapel to the nearest tree and broke off a branch with plenty of leaves. This would serve as a make-shift broom. Then he returned to the chapel and set about the task of cleaning it. For a time he toiled away on his hands and knees, unaware that he was being watched.

A group of people had gathered by the chapel door. They were surprised to see such unusual activity in this neglected church. Damien was interrupted in his labours by a knock on the door and, on going to see who it was, saw a man standing in front of some other people. He was holding some fruit which he offered to the priest.

"I am a Christian," said the man. "And I wondered if you were hungry and would care to eat this."

"Thank you, my friend," said Damien, coming out of the chapel. He told the people how glad he was to see them all. He promised them that the chapel would soon be ready and he would welcome all of them to the services.

As he worked in the chapel, another man entered

with an armful of flowers. These Damien arranged carefully. At last after more than four hours of hard work, he was able to step back and look with pride at the little chapel. He was weary with exertion but happy to see a chapel that was clean and beautiful with flowers. While he was standing there, a procession approached the chapel.

Few of the lepers survived more than four years, once they had been sent to Molokai. As Damien looked at the little group of people, he realized that it was a funeral procession. Four of the lepers were carrying a makeshift coffin and they asked if he would conduct the funeral ceremony. Damien agreed to do so and then accompanied them to the primitive burial ground.

After the burial, his thoughts were interrupted by a touch on his arm and he saw an old woman looking pleadingly into his face. She was breathless for she had been hurrying to catch up with the young priest. Although her face was very wrinkled with the years, she was not a leper. Damien smiled at her and held her arm to give support.

"What can I do for you?" he enquired.

"Will you please help me?" she asked, her poor old face looking desperately troubled.

"I am proud to be able to help anyone," he replied.

"My son is very ill and I am afraid that he may be dying," she said. "Could you please come to him?"

Damien followed the woman to a tumbledown

hovel. He had already seen dreadful cases of leprosy but this was to be the worst. The dwelling was little more than a heap of branches with a roof so full of holes that the rain had poured through, turning the floor into a quagmire. A young man was lying on some dirty rush mats. The old lady was so overcome that she could only wait in tears outside, while Damien knelt by her son. He administered the last sacraments and promised the old woman that he would baptize her the next day.

Damien was desperately tired and now wondered where he could sleep. He had no house for he had been too busy even to make one of leaves. Then he noticed the shadowy shape of a pandanus tree, sometimes called a puhala. He knew that it might be sheltering ants, scorpions and mosquitoes but at least it would provide some shelter if it rained. So he sat underneath it, leaned back against the tree trunk and lit his pipe. When his pipe went out, he put it by his side, placed his old broad-brimmed straw hat on his head and tried to sleep.

It was difficult for there was too much noise coming from the homes of the lepers. Some of them had been drinking an intoxicating liquor called ki, made from the roots of a local mountain plant. Then he could see two men fighting and, weary though he was, he went to them and forced them apart. Damien was very strong and the men, although scowling, went back to bed, leaving the priest to sleep under the pandanus tree.

The poor woman he was going to baptize died the next day. She was buried next to her son in the rough fenceless cemetery that was the last resting-place for all the lepers that came to Molokai. Damien spoke again to the men that had been fighting. One of them tried to strike him but he held his wrist so that he could not move. Many of the lepers were to remain unfriendly and suspicious for some time.

St Philomena's was a daily meeting place for the lepers. Damien encouraged them to sing, and arranged religious processions that were enjoyed by everyone. He soon had a band of willing helpers to keep the chapel in good repair. The joy of doing useful work for someone who obviously appreciated their efforts had been an unknown thing to them. Now they had a strong, young priest who cared passionately in every way. He talked with them, and prayed with them, giving them confidence that here at last was a friend they could trust and love.

In a letter to his Provincial, Father Modeste, Damien wrote at the end of his second day in Molokai, "I am willing to devote my life to the leprosy victims. It is absolutely necessary for a priest to remain here." Father Modeste had given Damien the option of having only a temporary stay with the lepers. Now after only two days, he had made up his mind that helping the lepers was to be his life's work. It was to be his way of living the Gospel.

3

"No greater love..."

Damien knew what it was to work hard, from his childhood years on. From his early years, he had also been drawn to the things of God. How he had loved those stories about the saints which his mother had related beside the fire in the kitchen of their home, with the shining pots and pans reflecting the flickering light.

How he had enjoyed the quiet moments of prayer, in the village church or while looking after sheep in the fields near his home. From the beginning of his priestly life, Damien did not spare himself in his efforts to spread the good news of Christianity and in trying to help all those he saw to be in need.

Even before he set foot on Molokai he had shown courage and determination to reach all those who lived in the portion of the Lord's vineyard which had been given into his care. Wherever necessary, he turned his hand to carpentry in order to provide his people with churches.

He set up a small farm to supplement the meagre missionary income and provide funds to buy the necessary building materials. But, it was on Molokai that Damien truly became "all things to all men" (1 Cor 9:22), and he needed all his love of God, all his physical stamina, to carry out the work he faced there.

A few months after arriving in Molokai, Damien wrote to his brother, Pamphile, telling him that he refused his assistance to no one:

"Consequently, everyone, with the exception of a very few bigoted heretics, looks on me as a father. As for me, I make myself a leper with the lepers, to gain all to Jesus Christ. That is why in preaching I say, *We lepers*, not *My brethren* as in Europe."

Long before the disease struck him, Damien identified himself with his poor lepers. He was their champion: he fought ceaselessly for their rights. He was a father and friend: he was totally available to help them in all their needs, from lifting broken spirits to bandaging leprous sores, from organizing musical and sporting events to making coffins and digging graves.

Not that he was "soft" with them – he cared too much for that. He won the enmity of some by dispersing drunken gatherings, brandishing a stick.

Something of Damien's alertness to the needs of others is necessary for all who hope to hear the Lord say: "I was hungry and you gave me food, I was thirsty and you gave me drink, I was a stranger and you welcomed me, I was naked and you clothed me, I was sick and you visited me, I was in prison and you came to me!" (Mt 25:35-36).

The total availability that Damien gave to the needs of others went to the extent of laying down his life for them: "Greater love has no man than this, that a man lay down his life for his friends" (Jn 15:13).

Damien was in no way a social worker who happened to be a priest. He was a priest who cared both for the spiritual and material welfare of his people. The material care he sought for, and gave to, the lepers was part of his spiritual care. He wanted to lead them to God – and he could carry out this all-important work a good deal more effectually if they were adequately fed, clothed and housed.

Damien was forceful and determined. Not only did he resemble the Christ who knelt and washed the disciples' feet, he was often like the Christ filled with righteous anger – and that kind of anger was directed by Damien towards officials who, he felt, were too slow to act, too uncaring.

With his availability to their needs, Damien was to bring joy to the previously dismal, harrowing settlement. He knew how to make use of their love of music, colour, singing: a band was formed; there were religious processions. Those whose deformities did not prevent their participation took part in games and horse-riding. He was, above all, the lepers' priest and pastor.

His care produced abundant spiritual fruit. Writing to Pamphile, Damien said: "My lepers are very fervent. They fill the churches from morning to night, and pour forth their prayers to God with an ardour that would make some religious blush!"

Damien's virtues have already been declared "heroic" by the Church. He is one of those who have "run the race" with a wholeheartedness that characterizes the lives of holy men and women over the centuries as they live out the Gospel. That wholeheartedness, that availability to others for the love of God, is something that anyone can practise no matter how mundane or monotonous a life he or she may lead.

We may feel that we only have small things to offer to God and our neighbour. But a major story would have been missing from the Gospel if a small boy had not handed over his five loaves and two fish to the Lord by the Sea of Galilee.

Damien's life and work can fill us with admiration and astonishment. But, when he handed himself over to God in the religious life, his education was insufficient for him to be thought of as a future priest. Openness to God and availability to our neighbour are what we need in order to be and do fully what God hopes for from each of us, so that we shall hear him say to us, as he surely said to Damien, "Come, O blessed of my Father, inherit the kingdom prepared for you from the foundation of the world" (Mt 25:34).

In the following chapter we can glimpse some of the ways in which Damien became "all things to all men".

How did he do it? Perhaps the answer lies

in his words: "Without the Blessed Sacrament a position like mine would be intolerable. But, having Our Lord with me, I am always happy, and work cheerfully for the relief of the unfortunate lepers!"

4
A multitude of good works

One day, shortly after his arrival on the island, Damien was making his usual tour of the settlement when he heard angry shouts. Two men were fighting over an old tin. It contained the precious commodity of water.

The incident worried Damien and he asked everyone how they fared for water. He soon discovered that there was a water crisis. Some people fetched water from a stagnant pool a long distance away but those who were too weak were forced to beg and even steal it from their neighbours. It was a dreadful situation, for the impure water caused the spread of disease.

That evening as he smoked his pipe under the pandanus tree, Damien thought about ways of solving the water problem. Towering over the trees in the distance were steep hills which shut off his little community. There must be rivers and springs of water in those hills. Tomorrow he would go to search for them.

When he awoke it was still dark but he had no desire to sleep. He walked down to the shore and looked out at the sea shimmering in the moonlight. He stood for a time in quiet contemplation at the beauty of the scene and then made his way to the chapel. When the sun came up he was ready to go, accompanied by a couple of men and some boys.

As he climbed the hill, he was able to look down at the village. On his arrival, the rocky hills had looked stark and the vegetation scanty. Now he found the view beautiful. He reached the top of the hill and then began the descent into a valley. It was very steep going down and he dislodged stones which went sliding away from him. He went cautiously and found himself facing a deep ravine which cut right across the hill.

The ravine was nearly two metres wide. He knew he could jump the distance but a miscalculation would mean certain death far below. If he was to continue his journey he would have to risk the leap. So he went back a little way and then, running forward, he leapt to the other side without looking down. He landed safely and went down to the valley. There was no sign of water, so he rested and had his lunch of fruit and bread.

He referred to his map and found that he had reached the Waihanau Valley. It looked a fertile region and he decided to explore. As he came through some bushes he saw something gleaming before him in the sunlight. With a cry of delight, he ran forwards and, going on his knees, thrust his hands into the clear, cool water of a large pool. He had found a natural, deep reservoir, full of fresh water: ideal as a source of supply for his lepers.

He could hardly get back to the settlement quickly enough to tell them the good news. As he walked along he planned in his mind's eye how the water pipes would be placed in position. It would be a difficult task to find enough helpers, for most of the villagers had little taste for work, even though the results of their labour, in this case, would be very much to their advantage.

In the village was a leper, appointed Superintendent of the colony. Unfortunately, he had little status with the government, but Damien went to him with a petition signed by the lepers, requesting medical supplies and other things that were urgently needed. The Superintendent was reluctant to send the petition but Damien insisted.

So, the petition was sent but weeks passed and they received no reply. Damien became increasingly angry and in the end wrote letters to the Board of Health in Honolulu.

One day, a ship called the *Warwick* arrived at Molokai. The schooner carried some much needed supplies, including the water pipes. Damien gathered a party of villagers and after some argument he managed to persuade a few of them to help with the laying of the pipes.

The Captain of the *Warwick* was a Hawaiian named John Bull. He supervised the unloading of the pipes by his seamen and had a friendly chat with the Belgian priest.

"We have to fetch water from a long distance," said Damien. "Many of the lepers are too weak to do this, so you are doing us a great service in bringing us these pipes."

Captain Bull watched the lepers struggling with the pipes and offered his seamen as helpers. "We have block and tackle equipment on board," he said. "That will make an easier job of putting those heavy pipes in place."

Damien sat on the beach with the Captain and drew a plan in the sand of what he hoped would be the new water system of Molokai. It was an amazing story of hard work, devotion to duty and achievement that Captain Bull took back to Honolulu. After he had gone, of course the work had to go on with as many people as possible doing their share.

Day after day the people carried the pipes and helped to fit them in a long line that stretched towards the reservoir.

When he was satisfied that a section had been laid correctly, Damien would hurry off to help anyone in difficulty. The others were inspired by his cheerful determination and worked extra hard. At last they had the satisfaction of seeing the final link of piping enter the reservoir in the Waihanau Valley.

When Damien returned to the leper colony, he was met by the news that water was already flowing through the pipes. Taps were fixed at many points in the village and, from then on, it was easy to obtain good fresh water for everybody. As the people came to thank the young priest for this latest improvement in their daily life, he felt that his efforts for them had been really worthwhile.

Storms hung over Molokai and the pathetic shacks offered little shelter when the rain became torrential. One day the wind blew so fiercely that a hut was blown down. Damien went to see what could be done to help and, with several others, tried to get the hut standing upright again. As they worked, the wind seemed to blow harder than ever and at last they had to give up the struggle and seek shelter in the chapel.

Instead of the wind subsiding, it became worse until it had the force of a gale. The fragile walls of dozens of huts were blown down and even the chapel was in danger. People who were able walked to the shelter of trees but others could only crouch behind what was left of their homes. Damien worked tirelessly and did manage to carry some people under large trees. That night, when he slept under his pandanus tree, he was surrounded by his friends who shared the tree with him.

At first he had been horrified at the thought of so many homeless people. When the wind and rain had stopped, he inspected the settlement and noticed how much cleaner everything looked. The rain had washed away all the dirt and everything smelled fresh and pleasant. He wrote a long letter to the government, asking for help after the storm. Not only had houses been wrecked but the hospital which he had so much improved, was also ruined.

When the schooner, *Warwick*, came to Molokai,

he gave Captain John Bull the letter. The captain agreed to take the letter to the Board of Health but he thought it would be better if Damien went himself. The need was so urgent that only Damien would be able to get the immediate attention that was required. There were so many homeless people who required someone to be with them at this critical time that Damien was reluctant to leave them.

However, this time there was too big a task for one man to tackle alone. It was necessary to persuade the government at Honolulu that attention must be paid to the welfare of the people who lived in Molokai. The Bishop and the Mother Superior of the Sisters could also be asked for help. So Damien decided that it would be well worthwhile to make the short sea voyage to Hawaii.

"I'll come with you," he told the captain. "As soon as it is convenient for you to sail."

So, for the first time for many weeks, Damien left Molokai. He liked seamen and the sea and enjoyed the voyage on the little schooner. When he was not chatting to the captain and his crew, he was busy helping around the boat. It was a pleasant and uneventful voyage and, with a good wind to fill its sails, the *Warwick* reached Honolulu the day after it had left Molokai.

Damien went straight to the home of the Bishop and was given a sympathetic welcome, and promised help.

"The most urgent need is for timber and tools to rebuild homes for the people," Damien explained. "Many people will die if nothing is done. I long to see them in new, clean homes where they can live with dignity and pride."

"I understand, and as soon as possible I will start a fund to help buy the things you require," promised the Bishop.

At least Damien had made an encouraging start to his visit and he left the Bishop's residence full of hope. Unfortunately, he was not to be so well received at the Board of Health. He entered the reception room and gave his name to the clerk at the desk, and said he wished to see the President of the Board of Health.

The clerk looked up and down, and asked if he had an appointment.

"No, but my business is urgent and I have very little time at my disposal," replied Damien.

Motioning towards a small reception room the clerk told Damien that he would make enquiries. As Damien waited the minutes went by and still the clerk did not return. He began to walk up and down impatiently. Then opening the door he looked out and to his surprise the clerk was back at his desk.

"Have you delivered my message?" asked Damien. The clerk looked up with a pained expression.

"I told you I would make enquiries. The matter is being dealt with and someone will be along to see you."

Damien returned to the waiting room but as the time passed no one came to see him. He was unaware that his arrival had caused quite a commotion. The government official regarded him as a troublesome nuisance whose work on behalf of the lepers in Molokai reflected badly on the government efforts. On hearing that Damien was waiting to see him, the President sent a message to his clerks that they should do their best to get rid of him as quickly as possible.

After hours of waiting and argument with the reception clerk, an official was sent to Damien with a set of forms and handed them to an understandably frustrated Damien. As he had no appointment, he was required to fill them in, stating why he wished to see the President.

Another half hour was to pass before the official returned. He took the forms from Damien and studied them carefully. Then he placed them back on the table.

"You have not filled these in correctly," he said.

Damien could hardly believe his ears. It seemed that he was a victim of a conspiracy to keep him away from seeing the President. With new forms before him he painstakingly filled them in once more and signed them.

"It seems that your superiors have decided that I must wait before I am allowed to explain the needs of my lepers on Molokai. They will find that my capacity for waiting will be something to be reckoned with and that I shall not give in to such discourteous treatment," Damien said bitterly.

The official shrugged. Rules were made to be obeyed as far as he was concerned and in any case he was merely carrying out orders. Hour after hour Damien waited until they could see that no matter how long they kept him he would not go away. At last he was shown into the office of the President of the Board of Health. Damien found himself looking across a large polished desk at a plump, middle-aged man.

"Could you please state your problems as briefly as possible?" he said.

"I hope you have time to hear about the problems of eight hundred lepers who are living in squalor and have lacked food and medical supplies since the storm," Damien said angrily.

"It is a matter that will be considered by my committee," replied the president. "These people cannot wait for your committee. They need help now," said Damien, raising his voice again. "What hope can I give them when I return that something will be done?"

The President began to look annoyed at having to face so many questions. "I can make no promises," he insisted. "We will have to wait for the report of the leper colony superintendent. Now perhaps you can allow me to other affairs that are awaiting my attention."

"That is the trouble. You have no time for these poor people on Molokai. You should be ashamed to neglect your duty in this way."

The President was not prepared to hear any more. He asked Damien to leave and reminded him that as he lived in a leper colony, he should stay there, "If you as much as cross the mountains that divide the leper colony from the rest of the island, you will be arrested," said the President.

"I cannot and will not obey such instructions" Damien replied. "There are occasions when I need to see my Bishop and there are parishioners of mine who live outside the leper colony."

The President did not answer but walked from the room. Damien had spoken his mind and could do no more. He said goodbye to the Bishop and other friends and then returned by boat to Molokai. He told the people there that he hoped they would soon have supplies of timber to build new homes. Immediately, sites were cleared in readiness while Damien prayed that his visit had not been in vain.

His Bishop kept his word and organized a fund which realized enough money to buy timber. This was sent to Molokai to build new homes. The work of building gave the lepers a much needed, worthwhile activity and made them happy. Soon, where there had once been a settlement of dirty hovels, there stood rows of clean, whitewashed houses. Apart from Kalawao, there was a similar building programme at the nearby settlement of Kalaupapa which was reckoned to be part of the leper colony.

To encourage hard work and quick building, Damien organized friendly competitions to see who were the fastest builders. He would walk from hut to hut and from one settlement to the other, helping and urging the men to get on with their work. He always carried tools, so that he could give assistance when he noticed progress was especially slow because the lepers were too weak to do heavy work.

Apart from all the effort he gave to helping these people building their new homes, he somehow managed to find the time and energy to build himself a one-roomed hut, about five metres long and three metres wide. For the first time since he arrived on Molokai, he would be able to sleep under a roof instead of the pandanus tree.

News about the progress being made in Molokai reached Honolulu and there were reports in the local newspapers. People began to ask questions about the lepers and enquire what the government was doing to help them. Because of public opinion, the Board of Health arranged for a shipload of timber to be sent. From the Bishop and the Sisters came not only a consignment of timber but also supplies of clothing.

To cheer up his people, he included in his service as much pageantry and music as possible. He formed a band and a choir and both performed regularly. St Philomena was always crowded on Sundays and there was not always room for everybody in the little church. Damien asked people outside to stand by the open windows, so that they could hear the service and the music.

In a letter to his Bishop, he described some of the work he had to do for the lepers. "After the Mass and baptism I take some breakfast and then start at once on my way to Kalaupapa, where I have three different gatherings: one for the old Christians of the district who are not lepers, another for the sick residing near the landing place and a third for those who live in the prominent part of the settlement; these last are thirty in number. I have not yet had time to leave the settlement. The weekly visit of all my sick parishioners takes most of my time. Next week, however, I hope once more to visit the whole island, if my foot, which is a little swollen from a wound, is healed."

Food supplies were a problem as the lepers were unable to grow sufficient food for themselves and depended on the occasional visit of a schooner from Hawaii. One weekend, the weather had been bad and no boat had come. There was a serious lack of food and people stood around on the beach, hoping to see the sail of a schooner in the distance.

At last a boat appeared on the horizon and eventually anchored offshore. Small boats, loaded with fresh supplies of food, were rowed towards the hungry crowd watching on the beach. Suddenly there was a sharp gust of wind and rain began to fall heavily.

Within minutes the sea became an angry cauldron, tossing the small boats about like corks. To everyone's horror the boats capsized about fifty meters from the coast and the boxes of food were flung into the sea. The sailors hung onto their boats and, after some worrying moments, managed to reach the shore in safety.

Damien could hardly believe his eyes as he saw the precious supplies of food swallowed up by the see. Later the storm did subside and another boat brought boxes of food ashore. The amount was totally inadequate and the schooner's captain was given a letter to take back to Honolulu. In the letter, the government was asked to send more schooners at regular intervals as food was always urgently needed. It was to be a long time before the food situation improved. To help matters, Damien encouraged the lepers to grow some of their basic foods.

In Kalawao, Damien's main concern was the hospital. Some of the lepers shared his hobby of carpentry and it was to them he turned when he needed help in building a new hospital. Once he had talked it over with them the village rang with the sound of hammers as the new wooden structure rose on the site of the old demolished hospital. When at last the new hospital was finished, Damien helped the people carry in the beds that had arrived from Honolulu.

There was no doctor, so he had to take over some medical duties himself, with the help of his friend Williamson and their medical book. Damien had to personally wash and bandage the sores of the leper patients every morning. Others, who were fit enough, he trained to act as nurses.

During his tours of the island, he had discovered Christian people living beyond the hills that ringed the leper colony. These people were not lepers but lived in isolated areas with little opportunity to visit a church. Damien decided to take his church to them by making a small, portable altar which he carried on his back when he visited them on horseback.

Of course by going outside the leper colony, he was breaking the law. Letters arrived from the Honolulu Board of Health, threatening him with prosecution if he continued to travel about Molokai in this way. He wrote to his Bishop explaining the problem and suggested that a new missionary might be sent to Molokai. His duties would be concerned with the non-lepers only.

In 1874 Mgr Maigret sent Father Andrew Burgermann, who was warmly welcomed by Damien. Fr Andrew was surprised when he saw the bright colours of the church.

"Is this your church building?" he asked.

"Ah! You are puzzled by our church of many colours," laughed Damien. "Yes, this is St Philomena's. I had it painted like this because this people love colour and I want their church to be a place of joy to them."

"You have done wonders here," said Fr Andrew as he looked at the neat rows of whitewashed little houses with their gardens full of brightly-coloured flowers.

"Yes, we are pleased with our progress but much remains to be done. We need a doctor, more medical supplies and more and better food. My church is too small and must be lengthened by at least three metres." As ever, Damien was thinking of improvements.

Damien offered to build a church for Fr Andrew and it was agreed that he should stay in Damien's house while this was being done. Damien set off for the south side of the island. The climb was hard but nothing compared to previous journeys. When he reached his destination, he told the people there was a new priest coming to see them. He was going to look for a site to build a church for this priest.

As usual Damien set out to work alone, watched from a distance by the villagers. As he hammered away, they began to come nearer and at last a big man came forward and offered to help, explaining that he had been a carpenter in Honolulu. "If there is anything I can do for you, Father, give me a hammer, some wood and nails and I will get to work," he said.

Damien explained what he was trying to do so that everyone could hear. Soon, others offered their assistance and even the unskilled helped to carry wood and arrange it for their friends to saw and hammer. In this way the church was built with walls 14 metres long and 7 metres wide. A tower, 17 metres high, was added and the church became an imposing landmark.

When Damien was satisfied that the church was ready, he returned to Fr Andrew and presented him with the keys. The new priest was delighted and grateful for all the trouble that had been taken on his behalf. He had some feeling of regret, however, that he had been resting while Damien had toiled to finish the church.

"There is no need to feel badly," said Damien. "The journey has been like a holiday for me and the hard work has been good for my health."

So the two men said goodbye and Fr Andrew set off for his new church.

Although he was still alone at Kalawao, it was comforting for Damien to know that not too far away, on the same island, was a fellow-priest and friend.

While Damien accepted the many hardships he had to endure in the course of his apostolate to the lepers, he suffered greatly when it meant no contact with other priests, particularly as he liked to go frequently to confession, as he strove to overcome what he saw to be his weakness and sinfulness and come ever closer to the Lord. In his early days on Molokai, he had had to resort on one occasion to shouting his confession from a small boat to his Superior on the deck of a stream – strict regulations regarding the isolation of lepers did not permit the Superior to land. Later the law was changed.

5

Light and shadow

After the law was altered to allow non-lepers to visit Molokai, Damien hoped to be able to welcome more people. He had naturally been very disappointed on the occasion that his Bishop had not been allowed to land. He was delighted therefore when he received a message at the end of his third year in Molokai, stating that Bishop Maigret was again coming to see him. This time the Bishop would not only be landing on the island but also would like to stay for several days.

Damien told all his lepers that the Bishop would be arriving on 8th June. He said that this would be a very important occasion and it would be necessary for everyone to make their villages clean and tidy. It gave the people a chance to work with Damien on all kinds of useful activities. They planted flowers, cut the grass and decorated their homes inside and out. It was a delight to Damien to see how happy the occasion was making everybody.

On 8th June sure enough a steamer could be seen approaching the shore. By the time it had anchored and a small boat with the Bishop and his party aboard was being rowed towards the land, horsemen had lined up to form a guard of honour. Hundreds of lepers had assembled to cheer the Bishop as he made his way slowly across the stony beach. He was greeted by Damien and then taken to the village where they rested in Damien's hut. As they sat there, the Bishop praised Damien for all that he had done.

"I know full well the conditions when you arrived here," said the Bishop, "and I am aware of the wonderful improvements that you have brought about."

"There is still much to do," replied Damien. "We have no doctors and no skilled nurses."

He took the Bishop on a tour of the settlement. Whenever the Bishop had a word of praise, Damien always replied that still more improvements were needed. As they came past a group of huts a crowd of lepers was waiting. They had assembled to welcome the Bishop but they also wanted to pay a tribute to their friend Damien.

One of them stepped forward to make a speech. He welcomed the Bishop to Molokai and then added in gratitude to Damien: "He overwhelms us with his great care. He himself builds our houses and, when one of us is ill, he provides him with food and clothes."

Damien had not expected to be mentioned in this way and stood quietly listening, his eyes filled with tears. Later the Bishop was taken to see the hospital before returning to Damien's simple home in order to entertain his guests. It was a warm evening illuminated by a bright moon and a crowd gathered to hear music. Father Aubert Bouillon, a Sacred Hearts missionary, who had accompanied the Bishop, was very impressed by the brave way these musicians performed in spite of their sufferings and he later wrote of them: "The musicians had for the most part only two or three fingers and their lips were very much swollen with leprosy, yet they played with great success many different pieces and entertained us for two whole hours."

This sort of determination could never have been forgotten by the Bishop and Fr Aubert who continued their stay on Molokai for five days. During that time they visited every home and went to services in both churches. On the final evening of the visit, Damien sat with his guests talking about long ago when they had all been living in Europe.

Their conversation turned to the colony and Damien explained his worries about the many orphans. His great ambition was to build an orphanage on the island to look after them but to do this he would need many shiploads of building materials. The Bishop was not to forget Damien's words. When he left he distributed special medals to all the children and later, when he was in Honolulu, he did his utmost to encourage the government there to send help to Molokai. It took time but eventually it was to achieve results.

When the steamer came to the colony, many people again gathered on the shore. The Bishop said goodbye, stepped into a waiting boat and, with Fr Aubert, was rowed out to the steamer.

Damien stood watching and waving until the

boat was too far away to distinguish its passengers. Then he strode back into the settlement, his mind full of plans. The Bishop had left money and he intended to use it to make a start on an orphanage.

As always with Damien, he was impatient to put his plan into action. As soon as he had been able to purchase the necessary timber, Kalawao rang with the familiar sound of his hammer. Helped by his boys, he built a large wooden house which was made as attractive as possible for its young inmates. These were chosen from all the most needy cases: a very difficult task as there were many orphans in need of care and even the new orphanage was just not big enough to hold them all.

With the orphanage filled to overflowing, Damien went to the government agent and explained that he would need extra supplies of food.

"Cannot the needs of children be provided for by the adults in the village?" enquired the agent.

"The needs of the children here will never be sufficiently provided for but we can at least try to do something for them to give them a little happiness in their lives. Will you deny them enough to eat?" said Damien.

The agent had often argued with Damien who was always wanting extra money and supplies for the settlement. He had to account to the government in Honolulu for the money he spent but after many visits to him by Damien it was at last agreed that the children should have a small extra ration of meat from government supplies.

Of course, Damien was not satisfied with the meagre amount of food and set about improving the situation himself. He went out to the fields and dug and planted for long hours at a time until a large area of ground was sown with sweet potatoes. While he was busy with this work he wrote letters to the government, the Bishop and the Sisters in Honolulu asking for their support. His sheer determination to get what he wanted eventually attracted attention. Appeals were made to the citizens of Honolulu on his behalf. Money began to be subscribed to help the orphans of Molokai. Damien had completed an orphanage for the girls. Now with extra supplies of food and building materials, he was able to put up an orphanage for the boys.

These orphanages added greatly to the work of the already overburdened priest. He had to be both teacher and doctor to the children, besides continuing his duties as a priest and doctor in the village and hospital. As always, he trained as many people as possible to help in the orphanages but these things took a great deal of time. It was in fact many years before the orphanages were satisfactory.

From time to time, Damien wrote to the Bishop to tell him that some assistance would be useful. Fr Aubert had left Molokai in 1880.

On one occasion, Damien wrote to his mother: "I live all alone in a little hut: lepers never enter it. In the morning, a woman, who is not a leper, comes to prepare my meal. My dinner consists of rice, meat, coffee and a few biscuits. For supper, I take what was left at dinner, with a cup of tea, the water for which I boil over a lamp. My poultry yard furnishes me with eggs. I only take two meals a day: morning and evening. I rarely take anything between. You see I live very well. I don't starve. I am not much at home in the daytime. After dark I say my breviary by the light of my lamp. I study a bit or write a letter. So don't wonder at getting only one letter a year from me."

His time was in fact taken up with even more activities than those described in his letters. His church, his hospital and the orphanages, occupied his every waking moment. Apart from the letters from Belgium, he sometimes read a religious paper, otherwise he knew little of world affairs.

The way he drove himself to struggle on, when he was really exhausted, took its toll and by the time he was aged forty, he looked much older. His once handsome face was lined and tanned by years of work in the hot sun. He had been saddened by the terrible human suffering he had seen and his face showed that sadness. However, his spirit and determination stayed with him all his life.

In 1881 Damien's work received royal recognition. King Kalahaua of Honolulu was on a tour of the world. His sister, Princess Liliukalani, was the heir to the throne and during the King's absence she acted as his Regent. She had read of Damien's achievements on Molokai and, while she was Regent, she wanted to go and see for herself what had been done to help the lepers. In spite of efforts by the government of Hawaii to dissuade her, she saild for Molokai on the steamer *Lehua*.

Damien had never dreamed that he would receive a royal visitor, and when he heard she was coming, he began preparations to welcome her. A triumphal arch, decorated with flowers, was put up where the royal guest would step ashore. Every building, too, was festooned with flowers and the gardens were made extra tidy. There were daily rehearsals for the welcoming ceremony.

As the sun rose over the sea, hundreds of people were waiting on the beach for the arrival of the *Lehua*. Damien shared the excitement of the crowd when the steamer appeared with the crimson and gold royal standard, fluttering proudly over the mainmast. He went from group to group, reminding them what they should do as the Princess walked ashore. The children, too, were not forgotten.

"Don't forget to scatter the flowers along the pathway of the procession," he called to them.

He need not have worried. Everyone was thrilled to see a small boat from the *Lehua* being rowed towards them with their royal guest. There were spontaneous cries of welcome and then a great wave of cheering as the band started to play and the small boat reached the shore. Damien stepped forward to greet the Princess and, followed by her ladies-in-waiting, they walked under the garlanded archway.

The Princess was taken to a platform which had been especially erected for the occasion. She sat with her ladies-in-waiting and other members of the royal party. Then a silence came over the crowd in readiness for the royal speech. The Princess was so touched by the sight of these poor people and the sincere and warm welcome that they had given her, that she could not speak. She could only try to keep back the tears. At last, she turned to her chief minister and told him to speak instead of her.

When the speech was over, she was taken on a tour of the villages by Damien. She was interested to see everything and to stop and talk to everybody. One poor man struggled to his feet when he saw her but the Princess, seeing how ill he was, told him to go back and sit in his doorway.

"You have made your garden beautiful," she told the man. "It is a great credit to you."

As she walked on, the Princess asked Damien how a man who was so ill that he could hardly stand managed to look after his house and garden so well.

"I encourage the lepers to help each other. If they have no one, then I consider it as my duty to help them myself," said Damien.

"This you have certainly done," said the Princess.

They walked into the part of the village that contained the church, Damien's home and the cemetery. He showed her these places. The Princess was distressed by much of what she saw, especially in the hospital where many of the people were very ill and disfigured. She was shocked that there were no doctors and that Damien had to try and do what medical treatment he could with some help from the more fit lepers.

The Princess told him he had great courage to carry on under such difficult conditions. It was obvious that she could not understand how it was that he wished to stay in such a place year after year. For his part, he explained that this was his work and he wished to do it to the best of his ability. All of the people they saw around him were his parishioners and he was their priest.

"As they are your parishioners, so they are my people," said the Princess.

Her visit had been planned to last for about an hour but the Princess could not see all she wished in that time. In the end she toured the entire settlement and her stay lasted all day. By the time the Princess was ready to return to the *Lehua*, darkness had fallen. As she walked to the shore, accompanied by Damien, the people sang to her. Many of them held lighted kukui nuts bound in ti leaves. These added splendour to what was already a beautiful scene.

Damien thanked the Princess for her kindness in coming to see them. She replied that it had been an amazing experience for her and that she would do all she could to help. She turned to wave her final goodbye to the watching crowd and stepped into her small boat. As she was rowed to the *Lehua* she remained standing, looking back at the crowd on the shore.

"Aloha!" she cried again and again. "Those poor people: God bless them all and Father Damien."

For some time she stood listening to the distant voices and watching the lights of the torches, still held by many of the people. Then overcome by the memories of the suffering she had seen during her tour, she sat down and sobbed. When her boat reached the *Lehua*, she had to be helped aboard as she still felt very distressed.

There were journalists on the *Lehua* and they noticed her distress. The next day the newspapers were full of the details of the royal tour. Damien received great praise, being described in one paper as "the glory and boast of Hawaii". News of his work appeared in newspapers all over the world. Damien wanted no publicity for himself. He had even been annoyed when his brother, Pamphile, had published a letter from him in the Belgian press. Still, Damien welcomed practical help for the lepers and he hoped that, through the visit of the Princess, more help would come.

In Honolulu, Mgr Herman Koeckmann had just arrived to act as Coadjutor to the ageing Bishop Maigret. The new Bishop was received by the Princess when the leper colony and the work of Father Damien was still fresh in her memory. She told Bishop Koeckmann about Molokai and asked him if he would go there on a special mission to present an award to Damien.

So another distinguished visitor came to Molokai. He had to spend much of his time on horseback, some of the riding being quite dangerous as the Bishop afterwards wrote: "About 10.30 we again mounted our horses and in an hour arrived at the top of the towering mountain that overlooks the leper settlement. The time had come to risk our lives and descend the craggy face... loaded with our luggage, we started down about noon. This perilous undertaking lasted an hour and a quarter. We had to clutch on to trees and rocks, slide on our backs, avoid the abysses where a few weeks ago a whole herd of cattle had gone over."

The Bishop also mentioned that he could not manage his baggage but the strong Fr Damien carried it for him. They reached the foot of the mountain safely where they were met by about seventy horsemen and escorted into Kalawao to the accompaniment of music. There were more bands and special ceremonies to greet them on arrival and Damien was presented with the Order of Kalakaua by Bishop Koeckmann.

The Princess had written a personal letter to him as well as the official document enclosing the award. In her letter she wrote:

"I desire to express to you my admiration of the heroic and distinguished service you are rendering to the most unhappy of my subjects, and to pay in some measure a public tribute to the devotion, patience and unbounded charity with which you give yourself to the corporal and spiritual relief of these unfortunate people, who are necessarily deprived of the affectionate care of their relatives and friends.

"I know well you, labours and sacrifices have no other motive than the desire to do good to those in distress and that you look for no reward from the great God, our sovereign Lord, who directs and inspires you. Nevertheless to satisfy my own earnest desire, I beg of you, Reverend Father, to accept the declaration of the Royal Order of Kalakaua, as a testimony of my sincere admiration for the efforts you are making to relieve the distress and lessen the sufferings of these afflicted people, as I myself had an occasion to see on my recent visit to the settlement.

I am, your friend,
Liliukalani, Regent."

Damien was delighted and honoured to receive the letter. He liked the Princess and believed that she would be a good friend to both himself and the lepers. It was pleasant to be able to have the Bishop visit Molokai but he felt embarrassed when he had to stand before a large crowd and be presented with the royal decoration. Bishop Koeckmann placed the red and gold ribbon around Damien's neck and then read out the royal decree announcing the award.

Some time later the Bishop was speaking to Damien when he noticed that the jewelled insignia was no longer round his neck.

"Father Damien! Your award has gone," said the Bishop aghast at the thought that by some mischance it had been lost.

"I have it safe in its small leather box in my home," replied Damien. Then seeing the puzzled expression on the Bishop's face he added: "I thought that such a bright jewel was out of place on my old cassock."

"Father Damien the decoration is meant to be worn whatever the state of your cassock. Will you please wear it?"

Damien fetched the medal from his house and wore it while the Bishop was at the colony; when his guest had departed the Royal Order of Kalakaua was put away in its small flat leather box and never worn again.

After eight years on Molokai, Damien could look back with great satisfaction for although much remained to be done they had been years of great achievement. Alone he had struggled against lawlessness and misery. In 1881 these evils still remained in the colony but on a smaller scale. There were now two schools; the teachers being paid by the government in Honolulu. More and better supplies of food were being sent out and from time to time large bundles of clothing arrived.

Yet Damien was not satisfied. He wanted to see a large modern hospital staffed with doctors and nurses where all the latest knowledge concerning tropical diseases, especially leprosy, could be utilized. Side by side with hospitals he dreamed of special factories where the lepers could do work that would not be too arduous. He wrote letters to the government in Honolulu asking for money so that a start could be made on the building of new hospitals.

In 1882 Father Albert Montiton arrived on Molokai and for a time at least Damien was able to share the work with another priest. After Christmas 1882, Damien wrote to Pamphile:

"Our young people go through the village beating two drums, waking everybody up and shouting, 'Merry Christmas'. The weather is beautiful. At midnight exactly, Father Albert comes out of the sacristy with his altar boys. The church is well lighted, filled to the doors, perfect order. After the Gospel, the preacher makes a great impression on the hearts of my poor patients. Although he is rather old, Father Albert has learnt Hawaiian very well. It is about two o'clock when all is over. Everybody goes home happy and pleased."

At the time he wrote that letter all seemed well between Damien and Fr Albert. However, Fr Albert was well known to be a difficult man with whom to get on. Writing to the Bishop, Damien said that he sincerely wished to live harmoniously with Fr Albert but that he was finding it difficult to keep his temper. Notwithstanding the disputes and difficulties which arose between the two priests, Damien greatly appreciated Fr Albert as a spiritual guide and wept when he left Molokai.

In 1884 Professor Stoddard, an American who had been to Molokai eighteen years before, returned to see what changes had been made. He was amazed and delighted at all the improvements he saw. Of his first meeting with Damien he wrote: "The chapel door stood ajar; in a moment it was thrown open and a young priest paused upon the threshold to give us welcome. His cassock was worn and faded; his hair tumbled like a schoolboy's, his hands stained and hardened by toil; but the glow of health was in his face, the bouyancy of youth in his manner; while his ringing laugh, his ready sympathy and his inspiring magnetism told us of one who, in any sphere, might do noble work..."

That same year Damien was also glad to welcome Doctor Mouritz. He had always complained that the hospital needed a qualified doctor. Now, at last, a doctor had arrived and what gave Damien even more satisfaction was that Doctor Mouritz was to be a permanent resident. Sadly, Damien was soon to be one of his patients.

6

The setting sun

In a letter to his brother in January 1885 Damien mentioned that there had been almost no feeling in his foot for the past three years. In another letter to his mother and family he spoke of accidentally putting his foot into boiling water – and not realizing the fact until he saw the skin peel off. He was well aware that the loss of feeling was an early sign of leprosy.

When he told Doctor Mouritz of his symptoms, he, too, feared that it was the first sign of leprosy. Of course, it was not surprising. He was in constant contact with lepers in the hospital and he was always working alongside them.

He worked harder than ever, possibly hoping to drive any thoughts about leprosy from his mind. Going past the school one day he noticed one of the boys, Whitebird, and a sudden impulse made him go to the teacher. He explained that he had promised to show the boy something of the island on which he lived and he asked if he could be excused from school for the day. The teacher agreed and the happy boy returned with Damien to his home.

After they had collected enough food for the journey, they set off together in the direction of the hills. Damien knew that soon he would not be strong enough for such a hard climb. So this was his last chance to keep his promise to Whitebird. When they had climbed over the hill they sat down to rest. A ship was on the horizon but not sailing to Molokai.

"I wonder where that ship is going," said Whitebird.

"To Honolulu, no doubt," replied Damien. "It's a very big one and must have many passengers on board."

"How lucky they are to be able to travel while we have to stay here all the time," said the boy.

Damien took the boy down the hill and close to the sea but did not go as far as the non-leper settlements on the island. They talked about Honolulu and cities far across the Pacific. Then it was time to eat their lunch which they did with relish.

"What fun it must be to sail on a boat," said Whitebird.

"Yes, it is; but so are many other things. We may not have the chance to sail on a boat but we can make our own fun here. You could try making a model boat."

"When I return to Kalawao I would like to come to your workshop, Father, and do that."

"And so you shall; I will be glad to see you there and to help you," replied Damien.

They began their journey back to the colony. As they reached the top of the cliffs Damien looked back for the last time at the interior of the island rolling away into the distance.

Then he led the way down the steep slope of the cliffs until they stood once again on the edge of Kalawao. Damien was so exhausted that he went straight to his home and rested on his bed but Whitebird hurried to tell his friends about his adventures.

The next day Damien, true to his word, worked at his bench on a wooden boat for Whitebird. The boy came to see him later and proudly helped to add the finishing touches. Then together they walked to the beach and in a small pool the new boat had its first launching. Naturally Whitebird could not keep his new toy secret for long and soon they were surrounded by other children watching how well the boat sailed.

The popularity of the little craft meant that other children longed to have similar toys and Damien felt obliged to satisfy them. Instead of making useful articles of furniture he now began to busy himself making various wooden toys. These gave the children great happiness which was shared by the leper priest. It seemed as if he knew that he could not have many more years and wanted to share his last change to be happy with the young inhabitants of Molokai. Sometimes he joined in their games and it became a common sight to see him playing with groups of laughing children.

His leprosy made no difference to his daily routine: he continued to work as hard as ever. If anything, he did even more than before and his manner was more relaxed as if a great burden of worry had been lifted from his shoulders. Where he had sometimes been serious and abrupt he was now more inclined to smile and be ready with a joke. He felt he should have official confirmation that he had the disease and when a German physician, named Doctor Arning, came to Molokai, Damien decided to consult him.

Doctor Arning had heard of the great work done for the lepers by Damien and was eager to meet the priest. As the doctor's boat came towards the shore Damien stood waiting for him. The doctor walked towards him with outstretched hand and the two men met on the beach.

"I am delighted to meet you, Father Damien," said the doctor.

Damien smiled but made no attempt to shake hands with the doctor. There were a few confused seconds while the doctor stood with his hand outstretched in greeting with Damien apparently unaware of the friendly gesture. They walked up the beach towards the village, with Doctor Arning feeling unhappy that he did not appear to be welcome to the settlement.

"I'm sorry I did not shake your hand," said Damien. "You see, I think I have contracted leprosy and I did not want to put you at risk."

The doctor was so shocked on hearing this that he could think of nothing to say in reply. They made their way to Damien's house and the priest requested that perhaps his guest would now give him his opinion as to whether he was a leper or not.

Doctor Arning carried out a careful medical examination and at the end of it he faced the priest. It was obvious from the doctor's grave expression that the news was bad.

"I cannot bear to tell you this but what you suspected is true. It distresses me greatly to have to tell you that you are a leper."

It was as Damien had expected and he took the news calmly. "Do not be distressed on my account," he said. "I only hope that I will be spared to continue my work here for some time to come."

"There has been much study of the disease," replied Doctor Arning. "The Norwegian scientist, Hansen, has discovered the bacteria of leprosy and doctors all over the world are trying to find a cure."

Bishop Koeckmann heard that Damien had leprosy although there had been no mention of this in their correspondence. To make sure if the rumours were true the Bishop wrote to Damien and asked him to come to Honolulu. The reply, when it came, revealed that the rumours had been true. Damien wrote, "I cannot come for leprosy has attacked me. There are signs of it on my left cheek and ear, and my eyebrows are beginning to fall. I have no doubt whatever about the nature of my illness, but I am calm and resigned and very happy in the midst of my people."

When the Bishop read this letter he was very concerned. Since November 1883 there had been a brave group of nuns headed by Mother Marianne Kopp who worked in the leper hospital at Honolulu. A Japanese doctor named Goto, a specialist in leprosy, had come to the hospital and introduced a special treatment of hot baths with medicine. Damien, after much pleading, obtained permission from his Superior to go to Honolulu for treatment.

The leprosy had discoloured his complexion and made his ears and nose swollen. He knew that there was little chance of his being cured but he was determined that before long he would be back. Before he sailed he had promised his parishioners that he would never forsake them and that he would return to them before many weeks had passed.

When the nuns at the hospital heard that Damien was coming to them as a patient they were very excited. They had read about him when they had been in American and he was their hero. To them it was a privilege to be able to nurse such a man and they did their utmost to make sure he would be as happy and as comfortable as possible in their care.

His room was scrubbed clean and whitewashed and Mother Marianne hung her own crucifix on the wall. The sisters placed pictures and flowers in the room; everything was done with loving care.

Sister Antonella was finishing making his bed up when Sister Leopolda Burns came hurrying into the room. She was in tears but her face was full of excitement.

"He's here," she said. "I have seen him talking to Mother Marianne."

"Why are you crying?" asked Sister Antonella.

"Because it grieves me to see him now when I recall his handsome face in the picture we once saw of him as a young man. Now it is disfigured with disease. He looks so tired and old for his years."

Before Sister Antonella could reply there was a movement at the door and Mother Marianne entered the room followed by Damien. He smiled at the two sisters but said nothing. With tears in their eyes they greeted him and then followed Mother Marianne from his room.

His treatment consisted of long hours in hot steam baths. This was followed by massage and injections of drugs. At night he slept between soft clean sheets, a luxury he had not enjoyed for many years. The rest and treatment might have proved more beneficial if he could have been persuaded to have been more patient and to be prepared to stay in hospital for a longer period of time. This was the last thing he wanted. He talked constantly of his lepers at Molokai and never a day passed without wondering if all was well with them while he was away.

"Instead of spending your time on me, just think what valuable work you could be doing at Kalawao and Kalaupapa," he said to Mother Marianne one day after he had been in hospital for a week.

"No doubt there is valuable work to be done

on Molokai but what we are doing for you now will enable you to return with renewed vigour and strength."

"I'm sure I will, but my stay here must not be too long," said Damien. "Not that I don't appreciate everything that has been done for me. You have all been most kind."

Mother Marianne shook her head wearily. Every day since his arrival Damien had reminded her that his stay with them could only be a short one and that both the sisters and herself were greatly needed on Molokai. As she was pondering on these thoughts Damien handed her a letter which he must have written with great difficulty as his hands were now very swollen.

"Please send this for me;" he said, "it is a message for my children at the schools. They will think I have forgotten them."

"They would certainly be wrong," replied Mother Marianne.

"No one could think about them more than you do."

"If you came to Molokai you would never forget them, I'm sure; the plight of those children is pitiful in the extreme," said Damien. "I hope that one day you will come to help them."

Every day he reminded her about the children until she talked about the possibility of going to Molokai with the sisters and found that they would be willing to accompany her if she decided to go.

When Mother Marianne saw Damien again

she told him that soon she would be coming to the colony with Sister Vincent McCormick and Sister Leopoldina Burns, although before they came they would have to get approval from the Board of Health.

At the end of his short stay in the hospital at Honolulu, he was seen off at the quayside by Mother Marianne. As he looked down at her from the deck of the steamer she waved and called to him, "You can expect to see some of us soon."

He waved back and shouted: "Please don't be too long before you come. There is not much time, you know."

As the boat moved out to sea they could no longer see each other. Damien stood for a while looking sadly at the distant coastline and listened to the weeping of the lepers on board who were bound for the colony at Molokai.

They had been parted from their families and knew they would never see them or Honolulu again. In his heart he too knew that this was to be his last voyage.

He breathed in the air and thought of the day many years before when he had first sailed into Honolulu as a young man from Belgium. His thoughts were disturbed by the voice of an American: "Father, would you care to share some wine with me in my cabin?"

Damien turned and saw it was the captain of the ship. It was the same captain who had once refused him permission to come aboard his ship to see his Superior.

"It is kind of you to offer me hospitality but you are forgetting that I have leprosy."

"I am aware of that and now know that to me you are the bravest man on earth and that it is my privilege to be your host."

Damien felt embarrassed by such praise, but the captain continued talking: "I have never forgotten that it was I who would not have you on board my ship to make your confession and now I beg you to forgive me for what I did."

"You are forgiven," replied Damien.

The captain went on to say that he was interested in religion but did not know a great deal about it. They walked to the bridge of the ship and there many hours passed as Damien and the captain talked together. By the time they had finished, the morning sun was coming up over the horizon and Molokai was not far away.

As Damien came ashore a joyous welcome awaited him. He had benefitted from his rest and treatment, although of course he was not cured. The leprosy had affected his legs by now and he walked very slowly but he was back on the island with the people he most cared for in the world and this made him happy. His small wooden hut had been kept clean during his absence and it was now lovingly decorated with flowers by willing helpers.

After he had rested he visited the village, the schools and the hospital and had words of encouragement for everyone he met. He might have had a rough manner with officials in Honolulu but with his lepers he had only words of kindness for he loved them more than life itself.

Within a few days of his return from Honolulu he was working harder than ever and it was difficult to realize that he had ever been away. After his day of work he would return home for his meal which he took outside his hut in company with the usual crowd of lepers who came to talk with him. They told him stories of their people that were legends handed on from generation to generation and sometimes they sang to him. When the meal was over and he was once again alone he would go indoors, light a lamp and sit quietly reading.

Sometimes he wrote home to his family or enjoyed reading their letters to him. He had been back from the hospital at Honolulu for some time when a letter arrived saying that his mother had died at the age of eighty-two.

Damien's brother, Pamphile, was still trying for permission to join him in Molokai, but to no avail. All his applications were rejected and at last he wrote to Damien saying that he thought he would never be able to come to the colony. Damien was disappointed as he would have loved to have seen his brother again but he accepted the situation and wrote to Pamphile:

"Our good God has fixed your residence in our native country, that your special mission might be to labour for the salvation of our family and others of our countrymen, as mine has been clearly traced out among the lepers."

As the weeks passed Damien's condition worsened. His face was badly marked and his hands were so swollen that he had difficulty holding things. He could hardly walk, his progress being painfully slow. He had always loved to go to the beach but the effort of getting there and back were now too much for him. An old horse-drawn carriage, given to him by a farmer living on the other side of the island, was used by Damien so that he could still enjoy watching the arrival and departure of the steamers from the shore.

One day, as he sat watching the steamer anchored off shore, he noticed a tall man standing in the small boat that was about to be rowed to the settlement. As he watched he saw the man helping to lift several large kitbags into the boat. This was strange, for if the man was coming ashore with such a large amount of luggage he must be expecting to stay on Molokai for some time. As the boat came nearer to the shore the man waved to Damien who had walked slowly down the beach to meet him.

"Good-day to you, Father Damien. It is a privilege to meet you," said the man.

"Welcome to Molokai," replied Damien. "But what brings you to our settlement with so much luggage?"

"My name is Joseph Dutton and I come from the state of Vermont in North America. As for my luggage, it is all I have in the world, for I am hoping to settle here on Molokai."

Damien stared in surprise at the man. He was

about forty-five years of age with an alert and intelligent face. Why should such a man at an age when most men are comfortably settled in life want to live among lepers. Seeing the priest's surprised and puzzled expression Dutton produced some letters from his pocket and showed them to Damien.

"These letters of introduction are from your Bishop Koeckmann and the office of the Board of Health," he said.

Everything was in order and Damien offered him a ride in his horse-drawn buggy. Joseph Dutton later described his arrival when he wrote: "We climbed into the buggy and were off to Kalawao... He was a leper in the advanced stages. I was happy as we drove over that morning. The Father talked eagerly, telling me how he had wanted to get brothers here but the Mission had none to spare. So he called me 'Brother', as though I had come to stay and gave me at once the full care of two churches. He was full of plans that morning, talking of what he wished for the lepers..."

Damien, of course, warned him about the conditions and the risks of working in the settlement and especially in the hospital. He also reminded him that he was not an easy man to work with and over the years he had achieved a notorious reputation for his sharp tongue. Dutton assured him that, whatever the risks and problems, he had made up his mind to stay and work in Molokai.

Dutton also talked of his own life. He had been born in 1843, the son of a wealthy American family whose ancestors had come from England. He had served as an officer in the American Civil War and had an unhappy marriage to a girl who had soon left him. Later he had been an American government official in Memphis but at the age of forty he had tired of this life and entered a monastery as a layman. After two years he decided that this was not his true vocation. He wanted to serve his church in a more active way. One day, after he had left the monastery, he was in a library when he read about the work of Damien in a newspaper. After a meeting with Professor Stoddard, he went to Hawaii where he received permission to go to Molokai from the King, the Bishop and the Board of Health.

"I am thankful that a man with your strength of purpose has come," said Damien. "You will be greatly needed here for, as you can see, I have leprosy and little time left."

After lunch with Doctor Mouritz, Dutton was taken on a tour of the two leper villages. In spite of the years of work that had gone into making so many improvements, the suffering of the bad cases of leprosy remained very distressing. Yet, although Dutton must have been shocked by what he saw, he showed no sign of wishing to keep his distance from the lepers. In fact he offered to help in the hospital, the orphanages and general building work.

So Damien and Joseph Dutton worked together

in the two villages. As the months passed, Damien struggled to toil as hard as ever. He was often forgetful as his illness took its toll and, in any case, was inclined to be untidy.

Dutton, with his past training as a soldier, was always there to see that all the jobs were done. At first he lived in Damien's house but later built his own hut.

Explaining the reasons for their friendship, Dutton wrote: "There were times when one did not care to be too much with Father Damien; that should be said. But there was love between us. That is not to say that our tastes and personal habits were the same. But I was firm with one resolve – to get along with everyone and everything. If my intimate association was longer than it has been for others, it was partly because I always saw him place in me the most entire confidence and I knew there was deep love in his heart, no matter what his exterior appearance might be. I used to be quite open with him in speaking of all these things; he, likewise with me; and this seems to have given us confidence in each other."

It was possibly Dutton's own character, however, that made the two men work together so well. Doctor Mouritz wrote of him: "Nothing ever causes him to lose his temper." After a year had passed, they were still working together and Damien tried to keep to his old routine. Dutton sometimes became anxious about him, noticing that he now had difficulty walking and there was always a risk that he would suffer injury through falling.

Damien's day had not changed all that much. He hammered away at a new extension to the hospital although the effort left him exhausted. As ever, his evenings were spent with his leper friends, sitting together as they ate supper. When Dutton was there, he would talk about his early days on Molokai when the pandanus tree had been his only shelter.

He told Dutton about the hot bath treatment: "Although I hated the treatment of hot baths that I had to have at the hospital, I think it did me some good," said Damien. "Of course it will not cure leprosy but it will bring some relief from the pain."

"Then let us build our own hot baths," suggested Dutton.

So for weeks they laboured at the construction of the baths. Damien's hands became so swollen, he could hardly hold the tools. At last the special baths were completed and the lepers were able to enjoy the treatment.

There was always so much to do that there was little time for leisure. Dutton was often advising Damien to rest but usually his advice was ignored. Then, unexpectedly, a letter arrived from Father Lambert Conrardy, a Belgian Walloon, living in the Rocky Mountains of North America as a missionary.

He had led an adventurous life and now, after reading about Damien's pioneer service to the lepers of Molokai, wished to come and join him. At first Bishop Koeckmann did not think him suitable and there was opposition to his coming. Father Conrardy was a determined man and eventually he was welcomed to Molokai by Damien.

It was wonderful to have the help of another strong and healthy man but there were to be other arrivals. The fame of Damien was now worldwide. In Chicago, an Irishman, James Sinnett, had also read about Molokai. He was a nurse and decided he could do useful work for the lepers. So he too applied to the Board of Health in Hawaii and eventually arrived in Kalawao. Damien immediately called him "Brother James" and asked him to work with "Brother Joseph" in the orphanage.

By the end of 1888 Father Wendelin Moellers, a priest of the same religious order as Damien, had arrived on Molokai. He was chaplain to the Franciscan Sisters who had come to run a home at Kalaupapa: Mother Marianne, Sister McCormick and Sister Leopoldina Burns. They did splendid work as nurses, taking over medical duties that had once been carried out by Damien.

They all worried about Damien who was now so ill that he needed the special help of Brother James. Damien insisted in trying to do something helpful every day as far as his strength would allow. He still ate with his friends, tried to do some reading and study and a little work but all activity now exhausted him. His once powerful body now looked thin and frail and his congregation were always anxious for him as he struggled into the chapel for the service.

Edward Clifford, an English artist, had read about Father Damien and was so impressed by the self-sacrifice the priest had made, that he, too, wished to go to the Pacific island. Clifford wrote: "The thought of doing so, naturally, gave me great delight, even though it seems to me that visiting Molokai would be the nearest thing to descending into hell."

It was not until the middle of December 1888 that Clifford arrived off the coast near Kalaupapa on a day of rough seas.

The boat had to go to Kalawao. Damien was there and able to welcome him. Immediately the two men were friends, with the priest calling the artist "Edward". Clifford described Damien as: "A thick-set, strongly built man, with curly hair and short beard, turning grey... he is now a good deal disfigured by leprosy, though not so badly as to make it anything but a pleasure to look at his bright, sensible face."

Edward Clifford came with an easel, and presents for the lepers. Especially useful for the hospital was the supply of gurjam oil which he brought. This oil was regarded as an excellent treatment for leprosy. Although he was sensibly careful about his contacts with the lepers in the villages, Clifford always made them welcome if they wanted to watch him draw pictures of local scenes and people.

On Christmas Day, Clifford sang with the choir

and in the evening he entertained all the people with pictures shown on his magic lantern. In those days there were no cinemas and the pictures that Clifford projected onto a screen didn't move, but his audience were thrilled by what they saw. They had little knowledge of the world outside their Hawaiian islands and enjoyed Clifford's pictures of great modern cities and snow-capped mountains.

On 31st December 1888 the artist had to leave Molokai. His visit had been brief but he had brought much pleasure to the people there and had done some interesting pictures. Damien and a crowd of people were there to say goodbye.

"Thank you for everything that you have done for us," said Damien.

"It has been a privilege for me to meet you," replied Clifford. "You can be sure that when I am in London, I will let the people there know of the work that is done here."

Edward Clifford took a Bible from his case and held it out to the priest.

"There is one last request before I go," he said. "Would you write an inscription in my Bible for me?" Damien's hands were so swollen that he found it difficult to grip things properly but somehow he managed to hold a pen at that moment. Slowly and painfully, he wrote: "I was sick and you visited me. J. Damien de Veuster."

Then, as Clifford's boat left, Damien was carried to some rocks on the beach where he stood leaning on the arm of Brother James.

Describing his last view of Father Damien, Edward Clifford wrote: "He stood with his people on the rocks till we slowly passed from their sight. The sun was getting low in the heavens, the beams of light were slanting down the mountain sides and then I saw the last of Molokai in a golden veil of mist."

7

"...For his friends"

On 18th February 1889 Father Damien sat down to write his last letter to his brother, Pamphile. He knew he would never see him again, for he was resigned to spending the little time he had left among his friends in Molokai. He told Pamphile that he was happy and contented in spite of his illness and he asked to be remembered to all the Community at Louvain and to all his family.

He had not forgotten the happiness that Edward Clifford had created in the leper villages. On 29th February he wrote to the English artist, telling him that he was seldom far from his thoughts and that he remembered him as one of this most beloved friends. He also mentioned the Reverend Chapman, an Anglican clergyman in London. Damien had corresponded with Chapman but had never met him. Even so, he regarded him as a good friend.

The Reverend Chapman had heard about Damien's work and had organized a special fund for the building of a new church in Molokai. He collected £1,000 and sent it to Damien to pay for the building. The money was soon put to good use and, ill though he was, Damien himself supervised the work and had the great joy of seeing the new church, which was able to accommodate a larger congregation, completed. It was the last time he was able to help in such work.

Every morning Damien went in his buggy to attend Mass in the chapel. Brother James was always close by, in case he needed help. He was often in great pain although the garjam oil that he used did bring him some relief and he was grateful for this gift from Edward Clifford.

During March his friends noticed that he had become slower and wearier in his movements. His mouth and throat were painful and when he tried to speak his voice was the merest whisper. On the 28th of that month he had to rest in bed all day. He was never to be able to walk again but his friends, especially Brother James, were always near him day and night. Although he was so very ill, Damien seemed content. Perhaps this inner happiness was gained from the knowledge that his great task at Molokai had largely been accomplished and others were coming to continue the work.

Right up to the end he had tried to do something every day that would be of help to somebody and bring them happiness. Among the last things he did was to make toys for the children in his villages. If he felt a little stronger, he would sit on a chair with blankets wrapped round him. Father Conrardy, Brother Joseph and Mother Marianne came to see him, as did all the people he had looked after for so long.

Father Wendolin heard his general confession

and they renewed the vows of the Sacred Hearts Congregation. On 1st April he said to his friends: "Look at my eyes. I have seen so many lepers die that I cannot be mistake. Death is not far off. I should like to have seen the Bishop again but God is calling me to celebrate Easter with himself. May he be blessed for that."

The next day he received Extreme Unction and seemed slightly better as he talked to the people around him. They marvelled at his cheerfulness but were sad to think that the end of his life could not be far away. Father Wendolin sat by his bed talking to him one day, when he noticed his cloak hanging over a chair and asked if he might have it.

"What would you do with it Father Wendolin?" Damien asked. "It's full of leprosy."

It seemed strange to the lepers that the priest who had always been so strong and worked by their side was now confined to his bed. They came quietly to see him to show they cared for their priest. Sometimes too many came and Brother James would scold them and try to chase them out but he admitted it was almost impossible to do this.

During April Damien's condition worsened and on the evening of the 13th he lost consciousness. This was the Saturday before Palm Sunday, when Father Wendolin had to go to Kalaupapa to take all the religious services. On 15th April, as Father Wendolin returned, he received a message that Damien had died.

The tolling of the bell in the church passed on the sad news of his death to the villagers. He was buried the next day under the pandanus tree where he had spent his first night on Molokai. In front of the funeral procession were the musicians with their band, followed by the Sisters and the coffin, carried by eight lepers. Behind them were the priests and at the back Joseph Dutton and James Sinnett with a long line of villagers.

Over his grave was placed a black marble cross, inscribed with these words, written in English, "Sacred to the memory of the Rev. Father Damien de Veuster. Died a Martyr to the charity for the afflicted lepers. April 15, 1889".

The pioneering work of Father Damien had become known in all parts of the world. His passing was mourned everywhere as news of his death was widely reported. In Britain, the Prince of Wales, later to become King Edward VII, spoke at a public meeting attended by Cardinal Manning and Damien's old artist friend, Edward Clifford. The Prince talked of the great example shown by the Belgian priest of selfless devotion for the welfare of others. He said that he hoped the achievements at Molokai would act as an inspiration to the people of Britain to help the thousands of lepers that lived in the British Empire.

As a result of this meeting, three suggestions were made: first, a suitable monument was to be sent to Molokai in appreciation of all that Damien had achieved. Secondly, a Damien Institute should be started where research could be carried out to find a cure for leprosy. Thirdly, a special programme should be begun to study how lepers were being cared for throughout the British Empire.

Certainly Damien would have been delighted to know that through his death lepers would benefit. A determined effort was made to put the plans into action. There were meetings, articles in newspapers and organized collections. A beautiful cross of granite was sent to Molokai. On the cross was a white marble tablet with the words: "Greater love hath no man than this: that a man lay down his life for his friends." The Damien Institute was founded and a great research programme started and the inquiry into the lepers of the Empire also was soon under way.

From reports that came after Damien's death, things did decline in Molokai. Father Damien had set a great example and his immense energy and sense of purpose inspired others to work hard and try to improve their lives. In a letter to Edward Clifford, James Sinnett, who left the island soon afterwards, wrote of drunkenness and a breakdown of law and order in Molokai.

It took some years for the situation to improve. Doctors came to the hospital that Damien had started and the children's homes were enlarged and staffed with teachers. Robert Louis Stevenson, the writer, visited Molokai and talked with people who had known Damien. From what he heard and saw, Stevenson left the island with a high opinion of the Belgian priest but a great dislike of Molokai.

Of Damien, he wrote: "It was his part, by one striking act of martyrdom, to direct all men's eyes on this distressful country. At a blow and with the price of his life he made the place illustrious and public... If ever any man brought reforms and died to bring them, it was he."

For forty-seven years Damien lay buried on the island of Molokai. Then, in 1936, his coffin was disinterred and taken to Belgium. A special service was held in his memory, attended by Leopold III, King of the Belgians, and many Belgian members of the government and parliament. He was finally laid to rest in the homeland he had left to become "all things to all men".

In 1956 Cardinal Van Roey, Primate of Belgium, opened the process for the Beatification Cause of Father Damien.

8

Damien today

by Felicity O'Brien

John Milsome has given us a colourful glimpse of the life and work of Father Damien. It is a story that has been told many times, and will continue to be repeated as long as there are people who appreciate heroism among their fellow beings. But, like all the images of holiness in this series, Damien is not simply a person to be admired but someone who has something to say to us today; a person who can inspire us to make the Gospel a truly living reality in our daily lives.

Damien's life and work illustrate admirably what the Gospel means when it talks about love. The word has too often been debased to mean a superficial sentimentality, or sexual attraction without a deep and lasting commitment between the people involved.

This is not the meaning of love in the Gospel sense; but neither is it a detached sort of altruism that scarcely affects the emotions. As Damien shows, to love is to care passionately not only for the eternal welfare of fellow human beings but also for their wellbeing in this life of preparation, for the fullness of life after death. If people view their Christian faith as somehow separated from the rest of their lives, they have not caught on to the reality of the Gospel. The charge has often been made that religion makes people unconcerned about improving the conditions of the poor in this life. Such people as Father Damien are conveniently ignored.

It would be difficult, if not impossible, to find anyone in history, or in our own day, who had done *more* than Damien to improve the material conditions of his fellow human beings. What was it that motivated him? It was not just humanitarianism. It was his deeply-rooted Christian belief – belief that each human being was of sufficient value to God that the Word of God came into a sinful world to save him or her, to make it possible for each one to attain limitless bliss in heaven.

The will of God, the thought of heaven – these were central in Damien's life. But it was because of them, not in spite of them, that he rolled up his sleeves and became the champion of those who had been cast out of society because of fear and disgust. The disease was quite naturally feared – at the time it was spreading rapidly and meant a slow death of an appalling kind. There was also the widespread belief that victims caught the disease through sexual promiscuity.

Damien's openness to the needs of others was something that developed steadily throughout his life. As a young man he was always a willing helper among family and friends, and it can have been no easy matter for him to respond to the inner call he felt to leave them and become a member of a religious congregation. He dearly loved his family and in a letter he wrote from Paris he said:

"Alas! the immense distance between us does not allow me to throw myself into your arms and to prove to you the feelings of love and gratitude with which my heart is so full."

But respond to the call he did. He hoped to become a missionary and respond to people's deepest need – for Christ and the Gospel message. It involved leaving his homeland and working for long periods without the spiritual help and support he felt a great need for from other missionaries. His generous spirit responded with even greater enthusiasm to the Bishop's call for volunteers for the leper colony on Molokai. He was not going into the situation blindly. While working as a missionary he had written home:

"Leprosy is beginning to be very prevalent here. There are many men covered with it. It does not cause death at once, but it is very rarely cured. The disease is very dangerous, because it is highly contagious."

However, nothing could fully prepare him for the sights and smells of the colony of several hundred lepers. He could have returned to his ordinary missionary work and no one would have blamed him. But faced with the appalling misery of the lepers there in the then nightmarish conditions, Damien responded with love – and stayed.

In order to help, he had first to overcome the natural revulsion and reactions to the conditions of the lepers. In the early days, he said: "Many a time in fulfilling my priestly duty at their domiciles I have been compelled to run outside to breathe fresh air."

Many of the lepers suffered not only from physical decay but also moral decay. Damien's plan of action was simple: "Kindness to all, charity to the needy, a sympathizing hand to the sufferers and the dying, in conjunction with a solid religious instruction to my listeners – these have been my constant means to introduce moral habits among the lepers."

People today are quick to admire a generous spirit – such as they see in Mother Teresa – but there is also a reluctance to undertake a life-long commitment. But, as Damien shows us, love in the Gospel sense means a commitment and getting involved. And it means undertaking that commitment and involvement without knowing precisely where they may lead us. It means letting the Holy Spirit have a free hand in our lives, putting the will of God at the centre and keeping it there even when the going gets tough.

Damien's attitudes towards sin and the sinner followed closely that of Christ. Those who fled as Damien strode angrily into their drunken gatherings overturning their alcoholic brews which contributed so much to the sexual immorality which was rife, knew precisely what he thought of immorality. But they knew too that this man bandaged their sores and fought for their rights. He did not just disperse drunken gatherings, he gradually dispersed the pall of gloom and despair that hung over Molokai. He drew the people towards the light of the Gospel, to a new self-respect, to an awareness of their continuing importance as human beings, to hope.

Damien achieved the balance that is sometimes needed today – of loving the person who has sinned – but never condoning the sin, never forgetting the Christian belief that Christ died because of sin. Compassion and deep respect for others cannot include a watering down of Christian teaching about right and wrong behaviour. But neither can the condemnation of sin include a self-righteous attitude. When Christ walked on earth he showed hatred of sin but limitless compassion for the sinner. He of all people, being the sinless Son of God, might have been expected to avoid sinners. He didn't. He ate and drank with them, much to the chagrin of his enemies. He stood between them and the self-righteousness of those whose reaction to sin was to feel not an anxiety to help the person but a wish to condemn, punish and avoid them.

Damien has lessons for us today on the meaning of love in the Gospel, on a spirit of generosity, of willingness to undertake a life-long commitment, of the fact that it is impossible for the true Christian to separate religious belief from concern and involvement relating to everyday life in the secular world, of the attitudes we should have towards today's outcasts of society, and towards immorality. But there is yet another lesson that we might learn and it is in his love for the Eucharist.

It was certainly the fountain from which he drew strength each day for his apostolate. His love for the Blessed Sacrament was clear when he wrote: "Without the Blessed Sacrament a position like mine would be intolerable." The Eucharistic presence of Christ in our tabernacles is a treasure of infinite value which can never be sufficiently appreciated by us. Some of the devotional literature from the past may not go down too well these days: each generation, each person, has to find new ways of expressing their devotion. But devotion there must be. We can never be reminded enough to honour Christ's presence in the Blessed Sacrament and to go, like Damien, with love and trust, into that presence.

Like so many holy people, Damien was a pioneer. Because of him attitudes towards lepers and the treatment of leprosy changed. That, along with the lessons we can learn from his life and work, is his legacy to the modern world. He paid a high price: the highest price – his life.

9

Words from Damien

"Oh, my dear mother and brothers, let us all live as good Christians, with the hope of meeting one day in heaven."

"Turn all your desires towards an eternal crown and do not be too anxious about temporal affairs. Let each one of us, in his own state of life, strive to amass treasures that we can take with us to the next world."

"Let us place all our hope, and centre all our desires in heaven, so as to prepare for ourselves a permanent home there by a Christian life here below."

"What are our young countrymen thinking of that they do not come forward with generous hearts to the field of battle and fill the gaps in our ranks which death and old age have made?"

"Without the Blessed Sacrament a position like mine would be intolerable."

"Truly the thought of the uncertainty of the morrow should produce in a soul most hearty contrition, but for us, Christian or religious, who look upon ourselves as exiles here below and who long for the dissolution of our body that we may enter our true country, there is, it appears to me, only joy and blessedness in the thought that each moment we get nearer to the last hour of our life. Then we shall hear those words of comfort and consolation, 'Come ye blessed of my Father, possess ye the kingdom I have prepared for you.' This is the blessing I wish for you and all those dear to me."

"We are in the hands of God, an all-powerful God, who has taken us under his protection... Take for your own this adorable will as manifested in the laws and commandments of God and of the Church, and in the voice of the priests Our Lord has given you, as the infallible rule of your life, of all your words and actions. This will it is which is represented in the Gospel as the narrow but tranquil way which leads to heaven."

"The more you detach yourself from the cares and good things of earth, the more you will feel that our dear Lord is the real treasure of the faithful. Turn all your thoughts and aspirations to heaven, and work hard to secure for yourself a place there for ever."

These quotations are taken from:
Life and Letters of Father Damien – the apostle of the lepers, edited, with Introduction, by Father Pamphile de Veuster. Published by the Catholic Truth Society, London 1890.

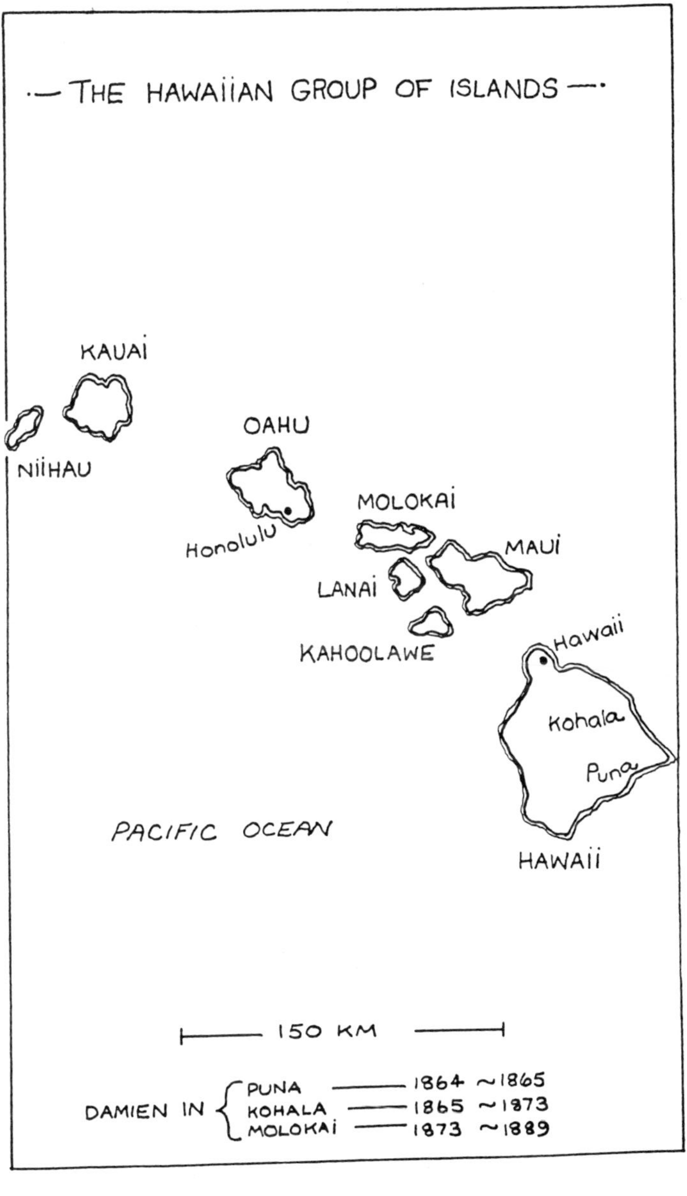

·— THE HAWAIIAN GROUP OF ISLANDS —·
KAUAI
NIIHAU
OAHU
Honolulu
MOLOKAI
MAUI
LANAI
KAHOOLAWE
Hawaii
Kohala
Puna
HAWAII
PACIFIC OCEAN
150 KM
DAMIEN IN
PUNA 1864 ~ 1865
KOHALA 1865 ~ 1873
MOLOKAI 1873 ~ 1889

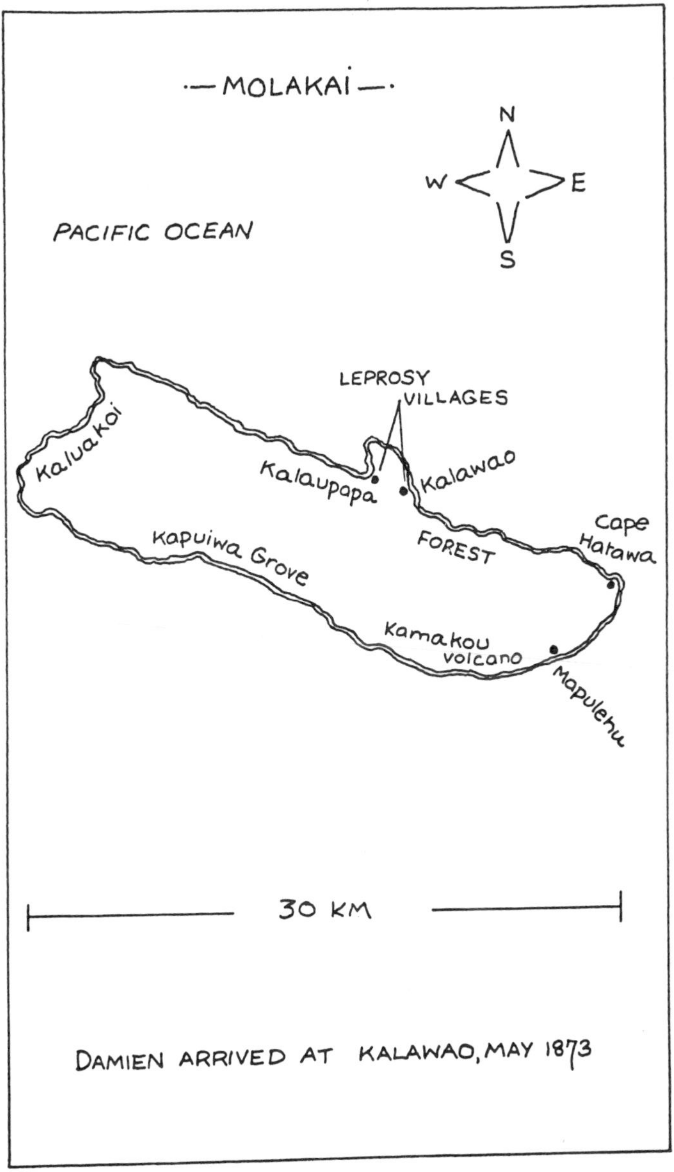
—MOLAKAI—
N
W
E
S
PACIFIC OCEAN
LEPROSY
VILLAGES
Kaluakoi
Kalaupapa
Kalawao
Cape
Halawa
FOREST
Kapuiwa Grove
Kamakou
volcano
Mapulehu
30 KM
DAMIEN ARRIVED AT KALAWAO, MAY 1873

THE CHEERFUL GIVER
Margaret Sinclair

by Felicity O'Brien

Margaret Ann Sinclair was born on 29th March 1900, in Edinburgh. For twenty-three years she lived an ordinary family life reaching out to people with her constant serenity and cheerfulness. She joined the Poor Clares in 1923, and died of tuberculosis at the age of twenty-five.
Margaret's holiness was already manifest among her contemporaries. She is an outstanding example and source of inspiration for Christians today.

FELICITY O'BRIEN is a freelance writer. For a number of years she worked with the Catholic weekly, The Universe, *and afterwards with the Independent Broadcasting Authority. She is presently Assistant to the Procurator for the Causes of the Saints.*

THROUGH THE EYE OF A NEEDLE
Frederick Ozanam

by Austin Fagan

A 20-year old student, Frederick Ozanam, and some of his friends, founded the Society of St Vincent de Paul in 1833. This was a time when the Church in France was the object of bitter hostility, following the revolutions of 1789 and 1830. Rather than involve themselves in political controversy and seek ways of reforming the world, the founding-members of the SVP looked for a more immediate and practical way in which to alleviate some of the poverty and suffering of those less fortunate in life.

The first part of the book is a dramatized account of Frederick Ozanam's life, while the second part presents reflections on some of his ideas expressed in his writings and in many of his university lectures and other talks. His influence led many others to follow him by seeking Christ in the poor whether they are spiritually, physically or materially deprived.

A book which reveals how Frederick's was a truly prophetic voice that still inspires many in the Church to speak out and act on behalf of the poor and the underprivileged of society.

THE HAPPINESS OF GOD
Holiness in Therese of Lisieux

by Susan Leslie

According to the best masters of spirituality a solid foundation of holiness is to give oneself to God in such a way that *his good pleasure* becomes one's joy. Therese of Lisieux had this magnificent obsession: *to see God happy.*
As she lay dying in September 1897, at the age of 24, she claimed that all her actions had been performed with that single aim. *Making God happy* was Therese's programme of life and holiness. This is the target she sets, even today, before the multitude of "little souls" whom she hopes to carry along her "little way" to heaven.

SUSAN LESLIE is a contemplative nun and lives in Oxford.

IMAGES OF HOLINESS

Series Editor: Felicity O'Brien, B.A.
Consultant Editor: Fr Paul Molinari, S.J.,
Professor of Spiritual Theology at the Gregorian University, Rome; Chairman of the College of Postulators.*

1. THE CHEERFUL GIVER
Margaret Sinclair by Felicity O'Brien

2. NO GREATER LOVE
Damien apostle of the lepers by John Milsome

In preparation:

3. THROUGH THE EYE OF A NEEDLE
Frederick Ozanam by Austin Fagan

**Postulators* promote the causes of candidates for beatification or canonization.